I0100189

MEN ON THE BOWERY

Sharing a pint of sweet Mad Dog 20-20 in the 1970's

A Research Report

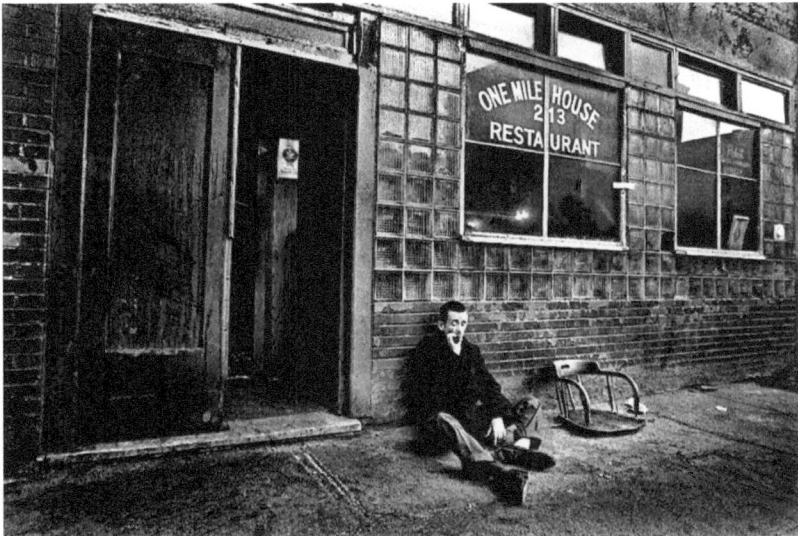

James M. Boles, Ed.D.

Copyright © 2023 James M Boles, Ed.D.

All rights reserved. No part of this publication may be reproduced, stored in a retrieval system, or transmitted in any form by any process – electronic, mechanical, photocopy, recording, or otherwise – without the prior written permission of the copyright owner. For reprint permission information, please contact jamesboles47@gmail.com.

Publisher: Vanishing Past Press LLC
Layout artist: Mike Miller

Front cover image:
One Mile House Bar, 1970's
Bowery Street NY, NY
Credit: Manel Armengol, used with permission.

Back cover image:
Two Men Resting
Credit: Joseph CA Mercurio

ISBN: 978-1-949860-03-0

Library of Congress Registration:

"History is not just stone, notable people, and bricks. It includes the reaction of those who were there and the community's ongoing response."

—Jim Boles

This book is part of the Vanishing Past Series published by Vanishing Past Press LLC. Vanishing Past Press is dedicated to the documentation, preservation, and distribution of works of scholarship and cultural importance with emphasis on under-examined or unexplored topics.

MEN ON THE BOWERY

Sharing a pint of sweet Mad Dog 20-20 in the 1970's

A Research Report

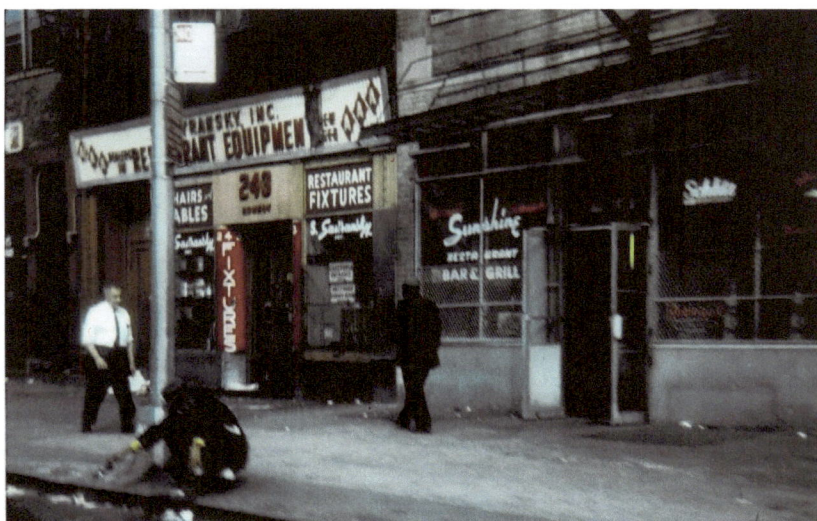

The Sunshine Bar and Grill, the Sunshine Hotel was above. 1970's.
Credit Brian Merlis-used with permission

James M. Boles, Ed.D., Fall 1974

Editor's Note: The exact language of this time and place has been retained for historical accuracy. No offense is intended toward any individual or group.

Dedication

To the Men on the Bowery:
Sammy, Tim, Larry, Pete, Dave,
and the unnamed who told me their story.

James M. Boles, Ed. D

Table of Contents

Introduction

My interest started with a walk through the Bowery of New York in the summer of 1974. The Bowery at that time was a fresh air mental health ward, a skid row nursing home, and a dumping area for the city's undesirables. It was like a small town where everyone had debilitating life problems. With institutions for the Mentally Ill starting to empty, many patients were discharged into the Bowery with its low-cost rooming houses and government-run shelters. Nothing was normal – you could walk just a few streets away and there would be students attending the local colleges; meanwhile, nearby on the Bowery, men crusted with dirt and blood were lying on the sidewalk – are they dead? How many, not one or two, but half a dozen. Should an ambulance be called? No, this was normal for the Bowery; everyone walked by, and the police drove by.

I remember one man with a bundle of colorful wires sticking out of his head – were they attached? They seemed to be attached. After this initial walk, I had to learn more about the Bowery and chose this study for a research paper. As I look back at my attempt to record the Bowery experience, at times it seems a little rough and naïve. However, it is a snapshot of a unique time in the history of this section of New York City.

What follows is a description of the Bowery of NYC in the Fall of 1974 by a new doctoral student in the Department of Family and Community Relations at Columbia University, New York. A few months before this, I was a live-in house manager in a group home for adults with severe mental illness, which likely colored my perceptions and interest.

This paper describes fieldwork in the Bowery of New York City in 1974 and gives the reader a snapshot of the 1970s Bowery. The language of the time and the streets is used, slightly toned down. No offense is intended toward any individual, organization, or group.

1

This study is about selected aspects of the lives of Bowery men and the environment they live in. These men reside in the immediate Bowery area and are usually described as "homeless" or "indigent" or, more likely, "bums" and "drunks." I will tell the story and let the reader form their own view of the men.

The study evolved from a curiosity about the area and its residents. From here, it took form from the people I talked to and the incidents I witnessed.

This book is dedicated to the men on the Bowery who shared their lives: Sammy, Tim, Dave, Larry, Pete, and the unnamed.

Chapter One – Beginning Field Work

Research while drinking Mad Dog 20-20 Wine

This study uses a research method known as participant observation. The simple definition of participant observation is researching a group by interacting with the members and participating in their activities.

The material is from discussions with residents and people who work in the agencies that serve them, the social workers, recreation personnel, agency directors, and my observations.

I spent over four months visiting the Bowery for this research. I ate, talked, drank, joked, sat, got bored, sat in doorways, visited the local bars, and went to clinics with the men. Most of the time spent in the area was in the hours from 9 a.m. to 5 p.m. on weekdays with a few evenings and weekends.

Initially, I started by going to the Salvation Army Booth House, a men's residence located at 223-225 Bowery Street, and talking to the people in charge. My primary contact was the head social worker. Through her, I was able to get administrative approval to be around the Booth House for the project. It would have been possible to be around the Booth House without this approval, as there were men who drifted in and out daily, some just for the inexpensive meals, but I felt much better with it. It also made me seem more legitimate to the men. I was often suspected in the area; many thought I was an undercover cop.

Working with the social worker, I met the men in the study. It was good to have a base of operations; my initial days in the area without one were frantic and I felt lost. The Salvation Army Booth House eased me into the Bowery neighborhood and gave me a place where I could hang out. The Salvation Army staff gave me a good basic orientation to the Bowery and the people who live in it. With my new knowledge, I could branch out into the surrounding areas, talk with the men, spend some time with them and visit some of the businesses and services they use.

Physically my main areas of study were the corner of Prince Street and Bowery Street, the Booth House, and the Mile House Bar; all events occurred within a few blocks of these locations.

The first days I spent talking to the personnel that worked in the area's other organizations, the Men's Shelter, and the BRC (Bowery Residents Committee). These contacts gave me a general feeling for the area and the different groups in and around the Bowery.

My typical day would go like this: Walking from Washington Square in the Greenwich Village section of NYC, I would enter the Bowery from 4th Street, turning right on Bowery Street, arriving at about 9.00 a.m. I would then go to the Salvation Army Booth House and eat breakfast.

I would stay in the Booth House cafeteria for a while talking to Tim, Larry, or Pete. Then I might accompany one of the men to an agency while they received services or go for a walk with them. On other days I went to bars with the men or moved to the bar's backroom to sit and talk. Often, I went alone to the Mile House Bar or the Majestic Bar. I covered most of the bars in the area during the study. Frequently, I spent the day on street corners or in front of the Salvation Army Booth House, hanging out with the men. I was at a loss at first on how to dress while doing the study. I finally settled on my older, worn clothes, not college student, nor 70's hippy like – which was very common, nor Bowery second-hand store goods. Most people told me I dressed like an undercover cop. I used to let my beard grow for several days. This made me feel better and more "in" in the area. I do not know if it helped. My wife, who worked close to the study area, tutoring a child who lived in a townhouse near Washington Square, would ride the subway to work with a somewhat shabbily dressed, unshaved man.

Chapter Two - Introduction to The Bowery

The Bowery Area and its Groups

By definition, the Bowery of the study is mapped as such: The principal thoroughfare is named Bowery Street. The Bowery extends from Cooper Square on the North to Chatham Square on the South. Side streets East and West are included forming the South side or East 5th street to the North sides of Doyers and Division streets.

Those are the physical dimensions of the Bowery. As for its social aspects: A typical description from the 1970s would include: "the Bowery area in the City of New York is occupied by men of all races and ages who present problems of homelessness, disabilities, mental health concerns, excessive use of alcohol and other antisocial behaviors."

The Bowery is also called "skid row." At this time in 1974 it is known primarily as the haunt of homeless alcoholic men, a region of rooming houses, streetwalkers, bars, liquor stores, helping organizations, second hand stores, and outlets for restaurant supplies. Walking down Bowery Street assaults one's senses. Ragged men gather, sharing a bottle of wine. Other men, in contrast, are neat, well-dressed, and lonely, living out their older years in poverty. This is the Bowery I saw and am attempting to report on.

Major Groups that are in the Bowery area

This is a listing of groups that use the area of my Bowery study. The groupings were discovered by talking with social agency workers, and residents, and by my observations.

Older White Men

This group includes neat, well-groomed men living in the Booth House or hotels and those found lying on the sidewalks in ragged clothes. Some are employed full- or part-time. Others are retired, some do not work, and most receive some sort of aid. It includes war veterans self-described as "never recovered," the physically handicapped, alcoholics, and the mentally ill.

The older white group and the drinking men may mingle. There is no clear definition between these two groups. There may be some mixing with older black men, who are friendly, but this is usually casual such as sitting together at meals. The Bowery is an inexpensive place to live, especially in New York City, and some men live there for that reason.

Older Black Men

They are middle aged or older. Some drink, some live in the area for cheap rent. They are a significant group, though not as large as the white group. It includes the infirm, mentally ill, heavily drinking, and veterans.

The older Black men and older white men informally interact.

Mentally Ill

These men are both black and white of all ages. They live in hotels, the men's shelter, or the Salvation Army Booth House. They are usually referred to agencies in the area from institutions and hospitals. They are a large grouping.

Black Homosexual Group

This is a young group, some living at Booth House, who hang around the men's shelter. There are streetwalkers in this group.

Jackrollers

I had no direct contact with this group other than the stories that the men would tell me. Their main hangout is in the city-run men's shelter, although some eat and live at the Salvation Army Booth House. Jackrollers in the Bowery are young men, often well-dressed, that prey cn older, weak, infirm, and often drunk residents of the Bowery. This group is feared by all the groups.

Women

There are few women in the immediate study area. Some are working at stores or agencies or living in lofts. There are streetwalkers on nearby streets, and on Bowery Street.

The women in the helping agencies have contact with all the groups. This is on an official level. As for the rest of the women the contact with the men is minimal.

Chapter Three: Sketches of the Men

These are neither case histories nor in-depth interviews. They are observations of the men and notes taken over a several-month period. With some men, I spent many hours, others only a short time; all spread out through the study.

Sammy

Sammy was one of my primary contacts in the Bowery area. We met in the Mile House Bar one Wednesday morning at 10.00 a.m.

Field Notes

Sammy

Met a man named Sammy who looked like Woody Allen, the actor. He had on an old suit, and a fisherman's hat pulled over his eyes. He was from New Hampshire and had spent most of the last few years traveling around and living in places like the Bowery.

He described it: "I did that sometimes; I would go into a town – Buffalo – I did it there. I didn't like Buffalo, didn't like the people I met in the bar, I usually went to a bar. The bar in Buffalo was too far from the bus station. In Boston there is a bar right across from the bus station, just across the street. Got blasted many times passing through that town. If I didn't like the people, I would leave."

Sammy, a white male, was 29 years of age, though he looked much older with heavy wrinkles and wear on his face. He is from a family of 14 children. His father worked in the "woods," a logger, and his mother in a shoe factory. Sammy can neither read nor write. He has held many jobs, from dishwasher, to battery separator at a junkyard (his top job). "Pay was good, best I ever had, $2.50 an hour and they didn't bother you. You just worked along, took your time."

Sammy was presently in The Bowery Project, a rehabilitation program for alcoholics. He was paid a small sum for each day's work as a floor sweeper, which was increased as he progressed through the program. "My final amount I'll get a day is about $15.00, how much is that a week, a month, a year? . . . Figure that for me, will you?" When I told him the amounts, he was astounded, well how much is $7020.00? Can I live on that?" We figured his budget and he decided that he could live quite well on the sum. He was living on $.75 a day at the time, his room being paid by the Men's Shelter, and he ate there also. He got very excited, "I can get a room at the hotel up the street, get my own room (he was sleeping in a dorm room), buy some good clothes, not real good though – don't want to look too good, keep living around here because it is cheap. Then I'd call home. How much money would I have again?"

Sammy said that he had been in the area for about two years. I asked him about his friends. "I don't make friends, no friends, just acquaintances. Friends can rip you off and do. Keep distance and keep safe that way. When they get too close, move on."

Sammy liked to visit the bars in what he called "rounds" often just spending the morning or evening doing this staying for one beer or coffee. He might visit one bar five or six times in one day.

The last time I saw him he was not drinking and was excited about setting up a shoeshine chair in the Mile House Bar. He was equally excited about the female bartender at the Majestic Bar.

Larry

Larry lives in the Salvation Army Men's Residence. He is in his forties and has resided in the area for two years. Larry and I met at the Salvation Army. We were introduced by the social worker. Later when I decided to do this type of study, Larry was one of the individuals the Booth House staff thought should be asked to participate. Larry readily responded and he and I left the staff office to take Larry's yellow sport jacket to the cleaners. "Shouldn't have bought it" Larry mentioned referring to the jacket as we made our way past groups of men passing bottles of wine or lone individuals laying out in doorways. As we headed toward Mulberry Street many people were out in the street – women, men, and children. It was 9:30 a.m. and the bars we passed' were filled with men – some drinking, some sleeping on the tables.

It was a bright cool New York City fall morning and Larry with his clean shirt and tie, polished shoes looked good and proudly strode to the cleaners, in marked contrast to the surroundings.

Larry then took me on a tour of his neighborhood. Down Prince to the left, up Bowery to the BRC (Bowery Men's Committee) – the former Bowery Gay 90's Follies Bar. We then headed up Bowery Street toward the Men's Shelter, a city run organization. As we passed, Larry said, "stay away – no good in there."

I asked Larry if he drank, "No, thank God, it's no good. Don't need that."

Many people talked to Larry as we passed – he knew and was known by many on the street. He pointed out several movie theaters that he frequented. We then parted that day, he went to the Salvation Army cafeteria, it was lunch time, and I took the train uptown to Columbia University.

Larry is known on the Bowery as being "not too bright." It is true, he cannot read or write. I encountered some Bowery men who could not read or write well. Larry is sometimes not aware of what is going on around him, he is naive and simple in his relations to the world. One morning I found him in a complete summer uniform of the US Army. Shoes, hat, khaki pants and shirt, polished buckle, and assorted patches and metals. Confused, I asked Larry if he had been in the Army. His reply: "I'm being a Boy Scout leader next Tuesday night and I'm getting my uniform ready." Larry had been promised that he could work with the Boy Scouts. From then on, he had some version of a uniform on until he had a complete one with appropriate patches and a red cap and scarf. A scout uniform with minor variations.

The Booth House social worker wanted me to see Larry's room. So, because she had to tell him something anyway, we went to the 2nd floor to his door and called for him. Larry proudly showed us his 3x7 room with no windows and wire mesh at the top. The walls were covered with nude pictures from magazines. From under the bed crawled a small yellow cat, obviously content.

A man bites Larry as he saves the dog.

Larry has made friends with a stray dog that hangs out in front of the Salvation Army Booth House. One morning Larry stopped a "drunk" from hitting the dog and was bitten by the drunk man, necessitating Larry going to the hospital emergency room for shots and stitches. When he walked out of the Booth House the dog would wag his tail and follow him.

The last time I saw Larry he was in full dress and was pouring over the pictures in his scouting handbook.

Tim

Tim was one of my main informants. He spent most of his time telling me about others and the Bowery, he was a good observer. Tim was in his 60s, he is thin, active, and intelligent. Tim does not like the Bowery area. He is waiting for his full benefits to start coming so he can move out and start "living again."

Tim has been ill for the last several years with cancer and other ailments. He was receiving cobalt treatments during this study. Because of his age and illnesses, he is unable to work full time, although he has looked for a job and did work part time as a dishwasher for a while. Tim has been trying to better himself by moving out of the area but is frustrated by his state of poverty. He tries to dress as well as possible and shops the local second hand stores for presentable clothes. I am convinced he will move out of the Bowery shortly. He is now a resident of the Salvation Army Booth House.

Tim is a former drinker now on Antabuse, the anti-alcohol drug.

One morning I went to find Tim after receiving word from the office that he was out of the hospital. I walked down the long narrow hall with its partitions of part wall, part screen at the top. I knocked. A suspicious voice answered.

Who's there?" I announced myself and he let me in – rather he let me stick one foot in the door as there was no room. Tim lived in a small cubical approximately 7x3, with chicken wire at the top, the walls were peeling, and the bed and chair took most of the room. Tim did not let me spend too much time in his room and hurried me out the door. I had the feeling that Tim did not want to be associated with that environment.

Tim saves men laying in the gutter.

When Tim sees a man lying on the street, in the Bowery or not, he stops and checks if the man is ok: "you can't tell if the guy has had a heart attack or what. I ask him, shake him, and see how he is. If he is not ok, he'll tell you. I've called the police many times for people. Just because a guy is not dressed up doesn't mean he is a drunk or not hurt. That's what people think – and just walk by." The men on the ground – you cannot tell what shape they are in or what they might do if approached – this was a very brave and honorable thing for Tim to do. He was the only one I witnessed checking on the men laying on the street.

The last time I saw Tim he was swearing about the agencies and the Bowery itself. He is full of hell and a pleasure to be with.

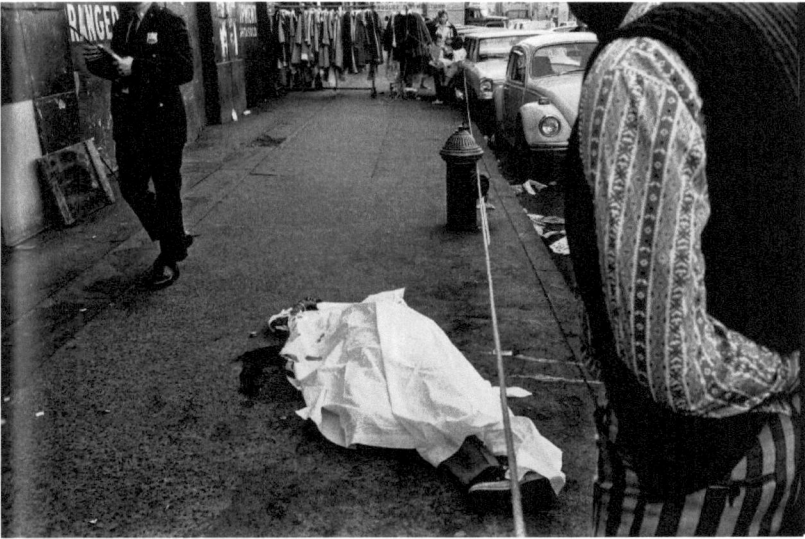

Man lying on sidewalk, Bowery 1970's
Credit: Edward Grazda

Dave

I met Dave, an older man, with a gaunt hollow face, only one or two teeth in the front, and gray skin, at the Booth House cafeteria.

I was eating breakfast when he said: "Got the world by the balls-on-top" His words were cheerful, but his physical appearance gave no clues to the reason for this joy. I asked him why he was so cheerful. "I get $700.00 a month from the Government, and I am on top of the world, yep, on top. Couldn't find my check and decided to see if it got sent to the Salvation Army, and there it was – so I moved in." As I resumed eating, he grabbed his stomach and proceeded to tell the story of his stomach removal operation – in graphic detail, showing his scar. "Yep, had it out 5 years ago. Doctor said it had to go, can't eat much . . . do you want this sausage or piece of bread? Here, eat this." I politely refused and went on to other subjects.

"How long have you lived here Dave?"

"Two days – got a bottle in my room."

"Where were you before?"

"Here, there, around, you know."

Every time Dave tried to talk, he ran out of air and was unable to finish and ended up gasping for breath.

Pete

Pete claimed that being so near death made him fearless.

I met Pete in the Booth House cafeteria. He was a friend of Tim's. A thin, short man who walked with crutches. His age, I would estimate, was about 40. He was born on a Native American reservation in North Carolina. He was raised in Pennsylvania, in the coal region.

He had been married, but his family lived elsewhere – "down south somewhere."

As the story is told and confirmed by others: Once at the corner restaurant that serves as a meeting place for the local prostitutes, Pete was approached by two girls. Women – "Come on baby – we'll take care of you – both of us." Pete – "It will take more than two of you. And it will cost you $20.00 bucks." Women – "Let's get out of here he's crazy."

Pete was sick, his legs and other ailments constantly bothered him. He claimed that his being so near to death made him fearless. "I am the one they send into the bathroom when there is a fight – I don't care – I am almost there anyway."

The last time I saw Pete he was sitting in the Salvation Army Booth House cafeteria, corner table – one can find him there any morning. As he said, "Jim, I'll be here forever, no one wants a cripple, the hotels won't let you in."

Chapter Four: Analysis of A Bowery Bottle Gang

Gatherings of men drinking are the first unusual thing you notice in the area. These groupings of men are called "Bottle Gangs," a name used by the men themselves. I first heard of the term from Tim, one of my informants. Standing, sitting, or lying-in doorways or sidewalks these groups come together for many purposes. The men say they form these groups for the purposes of "getting together, bullshiting, and drinking wine" – they also get together for the economic benefits, safety, and companionship. A bottle gang is a focused human cooperative organization to meet the participants immediate needs.

The Bottle of Wine – the heart of the bottle gang

Having Wine in the Bottle is All That Counts.

The center of attention in the Bottle Gang is "the bottle." This bottle is usually a pint or quart of port or other cheap sweet wine, Thunderbird, Night Train, Wild Irish Rose, and Mad Dog 20-20 were favorites. The main purpose of the gang is maintaining a supply of this wine, or "the bottle." The bottle must keep flowing to all the participants or the bottle gang is not working.

If money is available, then the problem is simplified.

If not, then action is needed. Members of the group are equally expected to share in the gathering of funds for the purchase. A member who does not participate in the fund raising must give up his membership in the gang, and it is clear, should not participate in the sharing of the wine. Even if a member does not raise any money, but has tried, he is eligible to drink.

The two primary means of raising money when no personal funds seem to be available is "bumming" from people walking by or in stopped cars. There are men, *known locally as "squeeze men,"* engaged in the attempted washing of car windows on Bowery Street.

The driver will often pay them something so they will go away. The washing of car windows is dangerous, the men are often intoxicated, and many are hurt, as they work directly in the traffic.

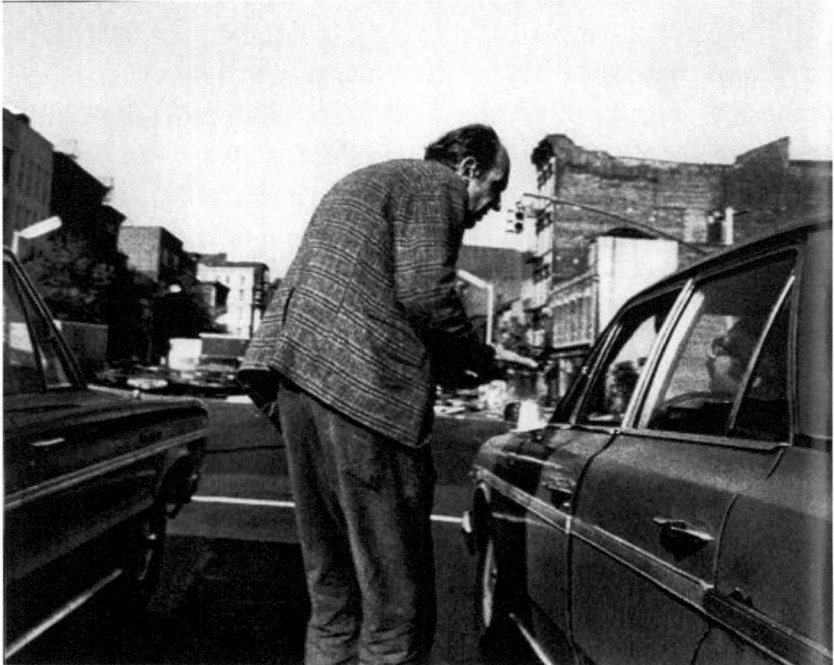

Man talking to the driver trying to raise money
Credit: Edward Grazda

These rules are often broken for example, a member might invite a non-member to drink, or someone too far gone might not be asked to participate in the fundraising but could have a drink. The breaking of the rules caused fights among the men. Sammy commented on this: "They are always giving someone else a drink – pisses me off."

The Banker: the money guy

Keeping the Wine Flowing

One of the key job slots in a well-organized Bottle Gang is "The Banker." A good banker will keep the wine flowing. The banker holds a unique position in that he must be trusted to collect the money as it comes in, from inebriated men, and bank securely the fistfuls of combined loose change and bills on his person. He also is usually intoxicated as he carries out his duties. He is further charged with "making the run," taking the money to the liquor store to buy the wine and most importantly coming back with the bottle. The banker is an important position in a bottle gang. Some men are always trusted, some never.

The Banker who did not return with the wine would not be allowed to be in that group again. As Sammy said: "Word would get out about him, the guys would get him."

Tim: "They will get the guy that doesn't come back, he could get hurt. He would not be wanted – no friends."

"If no one is trusted in the group then the whole gang would all go to the liquor store to buy the wine," said Sammy.

The Referee: stops bullshit arguments.

Another person of importance in a well running bottle gang is the man Tim describes as:

"A guy that can tell guys that they are arguing over crap, nothing." The problem of fighting seems to be one of the major drawbacks to bottle gang drinking. Besides physical harm, and halting of the drinking of wine, it creates a tension in the group that is not appreciated.

Sammy: "In the bottle gangs they are always damn fighting. No good. I don't drink in bottle gangs no more." The person that can contain the fighting helps keep the wine flowing and the group together, he participates, yet can remain objective enough to control the group. One advantage to keeping the group together is that one will get his share of the wine. If the group breaks up someone may take the bottle, or there may not be enough individual funds to buy a bottle.

These are not static groupings; they are subject to changes according to personalities and the personal money situation of the individuals involved. Shortly after "payday," the first of the month, there may be an ample supply of funds for the groups and little more than "splicing" (buying a bottle by chipping in for it) may occur.

Sundays, and after hours, because the liquor stores are closed, the men must go to the "Doctor" for illegal alcohol. This is an off-hour bootlegger of liquor who has increased prices because the liquor stores are closed, the Bowery has many.

A Bottle Gang

Most days on the Bowery, near the corner of Prince and Bowery Streets one can find a group of men some ragged, bearded, unshaven, dirty, smelling of sweat, sweet wine, and urine, others in comparison are neat.

Field Notes

I had observed these groupings for weeks and decided one day to approach this group. As I neared, I noticed a tall young man, about 35 and he did not look like he belonged. My first thought was that he was a reporter or a student studying the area. I knelt; the men were sitting or squatting, and introduced myself. There were three men. The young man, an older man with white hair, and a short Native American man. As I explained what I was doing in the Bowery, I was immediately asked "is it worth a bottle of wine." Later I did contribute a dollar to the cause. Mostly what followed was confusion for the first half hour as I attempted to find out more about why the men gathered on the corner. The men knew each other and were relieved of their boredom by a new member of the group – me. We were shortly joined by Bill, a bear of a man who had a loud guttural voice, his hulking body hovered above. He came over to see what my "deal" was, thinking that I had some type of "con" going. Bill brought little Jim Ray with him – a pug nosed former prize fighter.

My presence obviously changed the situation radically. I tried several times to discuss the Bowery and the men themselves. After several minutes I got the following mixed definition from the conversation, which I read to the men: "The Bowery, if you want to write about it you got to live it. You got to drink until you got the DT's, (delirium tremens) get kicked out of a bar then look for a place to stay, sleep in a cold doorway and wake up all screwed up and look for a drink. Then do the same all over again. That's the Bowery." All nodded their heads.

Several men talked to me privately and told me they would be glad to help in any way. While this was going on the ever-present bottle was being passed around. I shared its contents. The group broke up when the bottle emptied. I later found these same men in many more bottle gangs.

Chapter Five: A study of two Bowery Bars

I chose two Bowery bars for this study, The Mile House Bar, and the Majestic, both located on Bowery Street, New York City. From observations and discussions with Bowery residents these two bars were noted as being typical Bowery establishments serving a population made up primarily of Bowery men. There is a difficulty here in deciding what term to use in that in either bar one is likely to find a guy having coffee or a man that has spent the morning passed out on the sidewalk and staggered inside.

After the above-mentioned discussions with Bowery residents, I took a walk, observing the bars in the area, The Majestic, the Sunshine, and the Mile House, and others, and I then entered all the bars and spent a length of time in each, noting the dress of the men, their physical condition, health, and behavior – and the number of men sleeping on the tables. Most of my bar viewing took place from 8-5pm on weekdays.

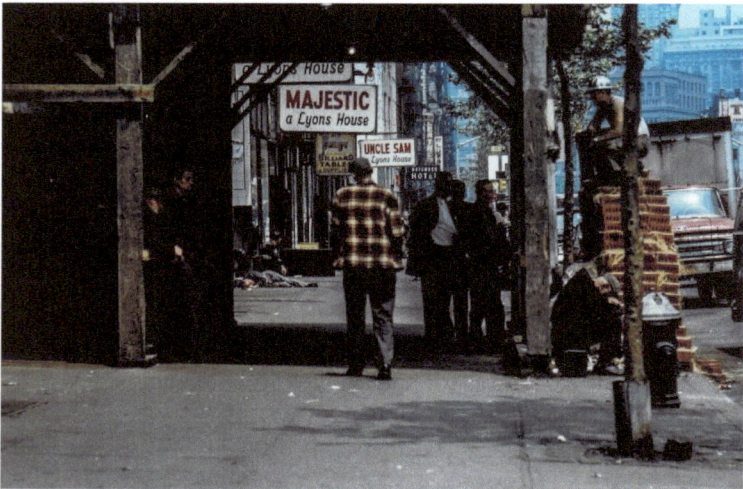

The Majestic, 1970s
credit Brian Merlis

Field Notes

The Majestic Bar

The Majestic is a long room with a bar to the right and tables to the left and rear. Men gather at the bar rail and most conversations are conducted here. The men at the tables are alone or in pairs, usually quiet.

All males, at the bar, all drinking, joking with a group of six with one of the two bartenders participating. Topics included women they had seen and alcohol.

The Majestic has the reputation of having a large night crowd, including the Hells Angels (they live on a nearby street). It also has the distinction of having the only female working in a bar in the area. As it was explained to me several times – she worked every night except Wednesday – everyone seemed to know her schedule. Sammy was the first person that brought these facts to my attention, his words on the subject were: "You gotta go there nights, that's when she's there. Biggest boobs I've ever seen."

Field Notes

I am at the Majestic sitting at the bar at 12:15 p.m. A man walked in and ordered a mixed drink. He then ordered a drink for his "buddy," pointing to a stool to his right. The bartender was confused, "What? Who's it for?" Just then his buddy walked in. They got his buddy a drink. Both of the men were dressed in new clothes, new black shoes, very new, and identical. One man was white, one was black. One said to the other: "Buddy do you have a cigarette for me?" The other, smoking a cigarette: "Get you own, get one from your friends. Don't: you have friends here? You said you had friends here. Get it from your friends."

"Well, I don't know, why don't you let me have one," this last said sadly.

"What about your friends, can't they give you a cigarette? Don't you have friends here? You said you had friends here. We came all the way down. You said you had friends." Shortly after this, they left, "buddies" to all appearances, one smoking, one not.

One Mile House Restaurant

The Mile House has a 20-foot bar rail, with a series of tables arranged in a long row with isolated tables off to the sides. Most of the men gather at the center row of tables for drink and conversation. At the single tables may be a pair of men drinking or as is usually the case one man sleeping with his head on the table.

The Mile House also functions as a hotel, a bar, restaurant and check-cashing station. It houses men upstairs ($60.00 a month) and feeds them downstairs in the bar, which has a food counter in the rear. It also serves them alcohol which is on a tab.

Field Notes

The smell. was overwhelming, vomit, beer, wine, sweat, and urine. Choosing to blend in, I noticed one of the patrons was drinking beer, a Schlitz split, 7 oz. I ordered the same. It was 9:30 a.m. There were 20 men in the bar. Some sleeping on the tables, their heads on their arms, some awake and drinking.

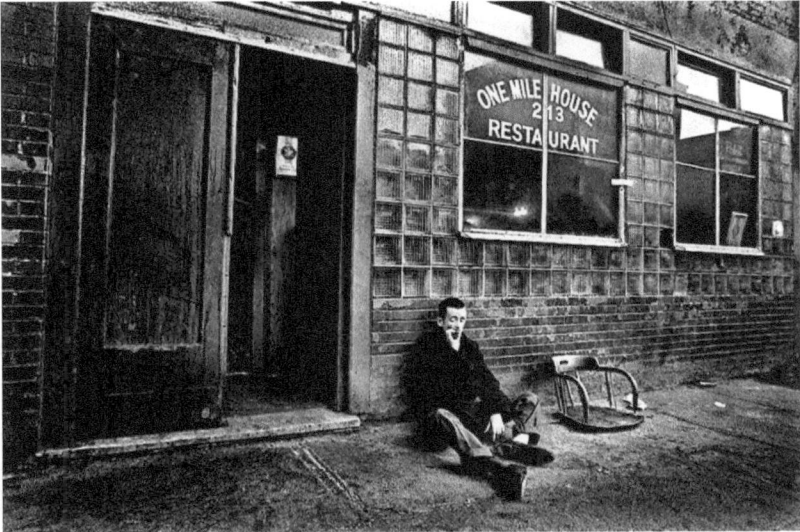

One Mile House 1970's
Credit: Manel Armengol

The guy next to me tried to get some money off me for a drink, he then tried to bum a cigarette. The bartender shooed him away. Shortly after I saw the bartender steal $16.00 from another drinker who was drunk.

The main gathering spot in the bar is the row of tables in the rear center. It is here most of the men sit, across from each other and carry-on conversations, one to one, or in groups. This seating arrangement allows a man to sit near another without really approaching him. It allows people that are not part of the group to join in the group. In any table setting there is likely to be one or more passed out or sleeping.

This bar had several distinct patterns of behavior. I first noticed that many behaviors were allowed away from the bar rail. One could be passed out on the table, fall on the floor, be crusted with dirt, vomit, and not drink, and still be allowed to stay in the bar room. Bumming of cigarettes and money was allowed here also. In contrast, the patrons sitting at the bar rail were generally better dressed, more alert, but not loud. No bumming of money or cigarettes was allowed. When one of the patrons angered the bartender, then he was usually restricted from the bar rail area, not the bar room. To sit at the bar certain rules must be followed. (Note: this was observed over a period of time, and many visits, with several bartenders.)

Field Notes

The bartender said to the man: "Get away from the bar – get away. I don't want to see your face at the bar." The man in question was staggering, drooling, and crusted with dirt and blood. His face and arms were covered with open sores, he had on hospital slippers. I later learned he was just released from the hospital. Although the man was physically in poor shape, he differed little in this respect from many of the other men in the bar. The fact that he could not stand up and carry on a conversation seemed to be the bartender's major objection.

The men sitting at the tables were generally staying for a longer period. Many spent the whole day in The Mile House.

If a man seemed to be delusional, not in reality or participating in an act repulsive to the bartender then they were usually scolded and sent away from the bar rail.

Field Notes

A young white man entered the bar eating an unwrapped candy bar with his hands. It was a warm morning. The man was crusted with dirt. He leaned against the rail and ordered a wine. And at 8:30 in the morning he ate the chocolate bar with his glass of wine. The bartender meanwhile was not pleased at the sight of this dirty young man eating a melting candy bar with his bare hands and was becoming more disgusted at each bite. As the chocolate melted and the man began to lick his fingers off, one by one, the bartender exploded, "Christ, what are you doing? Get back there and wash your hand off, you guys are pigs, get back there." The man somehow looked pleased at this outburst, went to the washroom, and shortly returned. His hands were a little cleaner. While he was gone the bartender talked to his partner about how happy he was that he had been able to get the guy to wash up.

The Mile House Bar is also a hotel and restaurant, and it serves many more functions than just a bar. It provides a place for the men to gather and get off the street. As one customer said: "I go there (Mile House) to put my head down, they let you." Because many of its customers are likely to be repulsive in that they are dirty, smell, physically ill, and intoxicated; the bar must tolerate many behaviors. The area around the bar rail belongs more to the bartenders and they establish this area's rules. The rest of the bar room is the area that allows other types of behavior, the intoxicated, the loudmouth, the physically repulsive and the sleeping.

Chapter Six: Payday on the Bowery

Check Day – "Misery feeding off misery."

I stepped around the man in the long gray coat as he slept on the concrete, his head resting in a thick puddle of yellow bile.

I left the Mile House bar, my stomach upset and my head full of what my eyes, ears, and nose had witnessed. Nine o'clock on Bowery Street, Tuesday, October 1, 1974, Payday on the Bowery. The checks come in.

The men are in line at the Salvation Army Booth House awaiting their checks. The air is electric. Jackrollers, who rob the drunk, sleeping, or infirm, filtered in looking for prey. As my informant Tim put it: "Misery feeding off misery."

In the Mile House and the other hotels, the boss may show up for the occasion, with his record book. Money is deducted for rent and board and loans (often at high interest, $5 for $7, $10 for $15). Some men elect to receive a part of their check each day, thereby rationing it for the month, they feel it is safer. Where would they hide their money? There is speculation about whether a man drinking every day can keep track of his money and whether he does get the full amount from the hotel. Most people say the men are getting "ripped off." Some men use the bar they hang out at for their mailing address. Men can receive full SSI and Veterans benefits self-reported as up to $375.00 per month.

Pay day and the days immediately following it are the time when the men get robbed most often. They have money and are often drinking heavily, becoming easy targets.

Field Notes

One morning last week (the day after payday) Tim answered his door to find two plain clothes policemen. In his words: "Dressed like you are, they showed me their badges. Very polite, said 'Sir. Excuse us but we are from the police department investigating the murder committed on this floor.'" So, Tim found out about the murder. "Á guy found strangled on my floor, killed him, they killed him. Right after payday, check day, they got him. He was 35-40 years old. "It's those Jackrollers who do it."

This was one payday in only a small section of the Bowery. Several men I knew were robbed that week, none were hurt badly, all had been mugged before, there were quite a few white bandages. It happens once a month.

Chapter Seven: Sex on the Bowery

On the streets, in the hotels, the agencies, the bars, there is a conspicuous absence of women and pairing of couples, straight or gay. This is what I was told and what I observed.

The few women that can be found on the Bowery are employed by the stores, agencies, or work as a partner in a family business. Most of these stores sell fixtures for restaurants and there was little contact with the Bowery men studied. The people in the stores usually stay in the store unless equipment is being washed on the sidewalk.

Another group that has little contact with the men is the Italian and the Puerto Rican women, from families who live up Prince Street and other nearby streets, who walk, shop, and live quite close to the men but neither bother nor are bothered by them.

The women who work in the agencies have the most contact with the men. These women are usually employed in a social service, recreational, or medical capacity and much of the interaction between these women and the men was of a professional nature as the women carried out their official duties.

There are women living in the few lofts in the Bowery area but their contact with the men is limited, not personal.

I talked to Tim about the subject: "Go up to Delancey Street and turn left. Streetwalkers by the park. Go up there and you'll get approached. I answered: "Yes, I was there last week at 8:30 in the morning and they were busy." Tim: "ya they must work in shifts. There's some there morning and night – they are there at 6 in the morning. Must be time and a half for the night shift. They go to the women's shelter and get cleaned up for a day or so then back out ... some women hang out with the drunks, drinking for companionship and protection, not much sex. Who would want them – they are both in bad shape." As for Tim's comments, I have seen many street walkers working this area of the

Bowery. From my observations, their customers were in cars and contacted the prostitutes, male and female, by pulling to the curb. I did not see any men in my group engaged in this activity. That is not to say it does or did not occur; but many of the men I studied having a great interest in drinking had excluded such things from their lives. The wine acted as a substitute for many things the men do without, such as sex and companionship. In Tim's words: "When you are drinking and have good wine – who would want sex?"

The director of the recreation section of the Men's Shelter, a resident of the area for many years, mentions that "the men don't have relations with women that might be available to them because their self-esteem or self-image is so low they don't or won't want to approach a woman until they are looking okay, clothes, money. And when they do go to a woman it is to a prostitute, because they can pay for the services and not risk rejection. If they don't have money, it's like them not having working male equipment, no money no sex."

Sammy had much to say on the matter: "These old bums couldn't get a hard-on anyway. A lot of guys go to the movie houses on 14th Street. That's where I go. The streetwalkers are scum, no good. I like to watch the women walk by on 2nd Street and Houston. Up there. Married women, ... I think, or maybe going to school. I used to live on 45th Street and sit out in front of the hotel. The street walkers, hookers, would talk to me looking for a place to crash. One took me out to dinner. Brought me everything. Drinks and everything. We ... you know ... just talked about things – nothing – you know. Never touched one, just talked. There's a bartender at the Majestic (bar). Big boobs, friendly. She talks to everyone, nice body, big (using his hands to demonstrate). Everyone goes there to watch her. She's friendly. talks to anyone, she kids around." What is missing from this description of Sammy's is the tone of his voice, the tone of wonder, of bewilderment, that a woman would bother to treat men, men like Sammy – so nice.

Another time: "Did I tell you about the bartender at the Majestic? About the two dollars? No, well I was talking to her, and I said, I'd like to squeeze your boobs, well, she said I could if I gave her a dollar for each one, so two bucks. I am saving my money and am going to do it Friday."

Sammy would like a relationship of any kind with a woman. He is frustrated by the women and relationships he views on the films and on television, and his present status. He talks of women as if they were an object he had viewed through a telescope or on film.

I see several factors as being important: The effects of alcohol and addiction on health; the effects of the physical appearance of the men and their ability to be with a women (or perceived ability); the effects of the men's state of life, poverty, low job status, (or perceived effects of this); the structural arrangement of the Bowery area and how this affects the amount of women in the area; the danger of the area; past experiences with the opposite sex; sexual preferences.

Most of the men in this study were often either medically involved, physically disabled or heavy drinkers by their own admission. Also, by their statements they were more interested in alcohol than women.

Because they were limited in their living area and the small section of the Bowery they lived in, due to factors of physical disabilities, and/or monetary restrictions, they did not meet many women, as there are few in the Bowery area.

Drinking, lack of money, poor grooming, a physical disability, may make them unattractive, in their own eyes and perhaps in the eyes of a sexual partner. If they do have relations, it is with a safe street worker, a prostitute.

The hotels and agencies in the area are primarily for men, discouraging women living in the area.

Many of the men have been married and had relationships in the past. They talk of these relationships, often with regrets, either being bitter towards women or blaming themselves for "screwing up too many times."

There is some homosexual behavior among the men, and there are homosexual prostitutes. I have noticed some individuals being openly sexual toward other men, this is limited, however, among the men I saw.

As found in this study, the Bowery men have little contact with women, other than casual meetings with store clerks. or women at the social agencies. No men I talked to have had any recent woman friends or recent relations with a woman. If one was interested in these matters (some because of alcohol, illness or just other interests said they were not) one was likely to collect Playboy magazines or go to movies on 14th Street. Those that did speak about women talked about the subject as if it were a distant sport in a foreign land.

These factors, low self-esteem, poverty, alcohol, and absence of women in the area combine to keep the men in a situation that is likely not to change.

Question? Where are the women who are poor, traumatized, alcoholic, mentally ill, disabled, medically involved – where are the women who have had a life similar to the Bowery man? Is there a Bowery for women? This is a large, complicated question not addressed in this paper.

Chapter Eight: Safety in Blending In

Safety in looking and acting like a skid row bum.

There are two things I want to do in this section of the paper. First to point out that pressures do exist on the Bowery, although it may appear the men are relieved of many of their responsibilities. Secondly, I want to show that to be responsible and safe in the Bowery may require actions that appear irresponsible and may cause behaviors that observers might think as irresponsible. The men adapt to the conditions and dangers of the Bowery to survive.

People I spoke to, who were not residents of the area often talked about the Bowery as if it were a paradise. The only place to be if you are a drunk, or a poor man. Providing one with food, clothing, and shelter, and other supports such as help with getting medical care and benefits with little stigma attached to being intoxicated or being a drunk. The Bowery can be an inexpensive place to live and can be seen as a living situation with few obvious obligations. Bendier in his book, *The Bowery Man*, can be interpreted as having a central theme that the Bowery is an easy way of life for the men[1]. *The Bowery Project*, a research project about the area also mentions, "... the investigator noticed many times the phrases, 'no one bothers me, free to come and go,' Additional questioning ... confirmed the impression that these homeless men are uniquely non-responsible."[2]

---

[1] The Bowery Man, Bender, Elmer. Thomas Nelson & Sons, NY 1961 or at end of book++

[2] The Bowery Project, Bureau of Applied Social Research, Columbia University, NY, Bowery Project – Summary Report, 1963

These thoughts are all true if one follows the thinking that the Bowery allows the men to drop many of the standards and norms they may have had, such as proper grooming, dress; public behavior, polite interactions with men and women, and this behavior is characteristic of the type of men that gravitate to the area. It is often called by observers the behavior of "drunks," or "people who don't care." It could be felt that the men ended up here because this is where this type of man goes.

To appearances this may seem so, but my findings show that the Bowery acts as a reinforcement for unusual behaviors, and in many cases supports them. If a man lives in the Bowery some release of pressure occurs, and a measure of security, when he has or obtains these "undesirable characteristics."

Field Notes

Pressure to drink

I talked to Pete today. I met him through Tim. Pete told me of the demands he was getting from the "guys" to drink even though he was a dry alcoholic trying to stay sober. "One guy asked me if I wanted a drink, then when I said no to that, I was trying to stay dry, he hit me over the head with the bottle. A lot of guys won't hang around with you if you don't drink. How can you spend time with guys you know if they are in bars or street drinking and won't let you just sit there?"

This could be of importance to men with few close friends and who are lonely, such as the men I met on the Bowery, and would especially affect alcoholics trying to dry out – quit drinking. The pressure to drink and the means to alcohol and social groups who are drinkers are readily available. The men had few apparent obligations that would be delayed or not met. They did have many boring days. Some would schedule things to do such as going to the Men's Club at 11:00 or look forward to a doctor's appointment or a planned talk with the social worker. The area bars such as the Mile House and the Majestic open at 8:00 a.m. to provide services to waiting customers. By 9:00 a.m. they are full of men. The primary means of diversion or entertainment is talking, preferably in groups, while drinking.

Looking Like a Bum

As for the "undesirable" characteristic of improper dress, one main cause of this is lack of money, and facilities to wash clothes. Another factor affecting dress is the high mugging rate of the area. If one is too dressed up one is more likely to be robbed, if one has good clothes, they will be taken. The men staying at the Bowery Men's Shelter and other SRO (single room only) rooming houses are instructed to, and know to, secure their valuables, this includes hiding their coats and shoes. No one wears a watch, although canes are often carried for protection. Every man I talked to had been robbed many times.

"Grooming" is affected by lack of proper facilities, being out on the street and visible during the day because of facility rules, lack of funds and lack of need to groom. Haircuts cost money. You never want to look too groomed – it is dangerous.

In contrast to this there are men like Tim and Pete, who are neatly dressed in secondhand clothes, but they know not to look too good. These men are not drinking and are more careful of their behavior because they know that if they look reasonably good, they are possible targets for mugging. They only go to certain locations and at safe times.

Many of the activities of the Bowery men are on display, easily viewed, and occur often on public streets. This is due to several factors including the rules of most hotels in the area requiring the men to be out in the morning for cleaning.

Only a few of the hotels have small TV rooms but most do not allow drinking or may discourage sleeping, often facilities are not usable and forbidden to those hotel guests who are on "tickets" (passes from the

Men's Shelter that allow one to sleep in a selected hotel). So those men on the street, laying on the sidewalk, sleeping in doorways may have a room nearby but are unable to use it or the facilities from early a.m. to afternoon.

The bars often will not allow all the behavior that occurs on the street, some for instance discourage "bumming" for cigarettes or money and sleeping on tables. The price of a bottle is cheaper from a liquor store, than a bar, which encourages the buying of a bottle and sharing it with fellows on the street, for all to see.

"Count your fingers" Anti-social hostile Behavior

In the Bowery you may witness anti-social, hostile, or withdrawn behavior. As a group, the men are suspicious, suspicious of themselves and especially of people they do not know. One of the Bowery jokes going around is "if you shake hands with someone, better count your fingers." "Count your fingers" is often shouted after a handshake. With the suspicion is much actual fear of others.

Tim has been mugged several times. When he goes out at night, he carries a short length of pipe.

Sammy has similar views of the danger of the Bowery area. Here are his suggestions for how to behave to avoid getting mugged.

"Don't walk fast, take your time, look in garbage (to show you are a resident of the area). People are watching all the time, cops and Jackrollers, look around, don't dress too well."

In spite of Sammy's precautions, he was mugged last Friday, when he got drunk.

The few months I was in the Bowery there were four deaths, that I knew of, the latest a knifing at the Bowery East bar. Many people I knew were mugged and injured. There are always a number of men with injured legs and cuts on the head, with the ever-present white bandages, the result of muggings.

The men living under the ever-pervasive fear may develop a deep distrust of their fellow men and especially of strangers. This truly seemed to be the case as relations between men were of a non-trusting nature resulting in what appears to be non-friendly behavior.

Sammy's thoughts on this matter were: "Don't make friends, make acquaintances, I never make friends some people might, I don't know, I don't. Friends might rip you off and they do. Keep your distance, you keep safe that way."

Observations of these relations showed that this attitude of Sammy's was essentially universal. There were few buddies that went around together but these relationships were often short with one partner getting mad and leaving for what might be considered a minor incident, or one going to the hospital. Most men keep to themselves but have several talking friends with whom they meet at the Booth House cafeteria, the bar, or the street. These groupings might occur at a regular time of the day, such as at meals, or after meals, few seem planned or arranged. It was also true that acquaintances were easily made. People I met only once were calling me their "friends," by the second meeting we were "buddies."

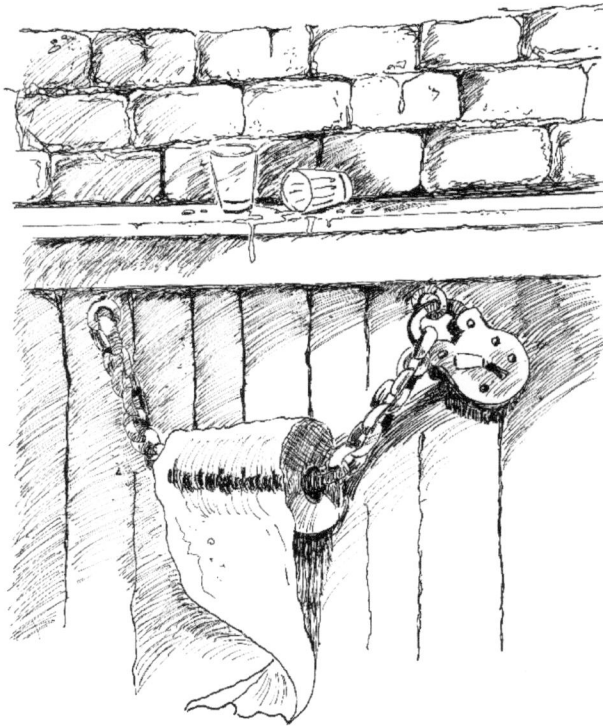

Image from memory of a Bowery bar men's room.
Even the toilet paper was locked down.
Artist: Paul Martin.

Chapter Nine: Summary and Conclusions

This study is about selected aspects of the lives of several Bowery men. Using participant observation research methods, I spent four months in the fall of 1974, in the Bowery interacting with residents. The men who were involved were uniquely different in their lifestyles and their view of life. Some lived in the Bowery because it was the only housing they could afford in New York City, some lived there because they were discharged into the Bowery from an institution.

The Bowery man is under pressure to behave in many ways that could be looked on as non-responsible or undesirable, such as drinking in public, ragged clothes, anti-social behavior, and poor grooming. It is often the need to survive in the Bowery that causes many of these behaviors, not the innate characteristics of the men.

The Bowery of 1974 has a large number of men living in states of poor physical and mental health and under conditions that are inadequate, dangerous, degrading and self-limiting. It is one of the areas that house New York's outcasts. Because of the large number of agencies and cheap living facilities available, men gravitate to the area.

It is as if the men are being maintained in this area of the city because it is easier to "treat" them if they are together. Which in many ways is true.

The Bowery is a way of life. A life of struggle, poverty, poor living conditions, danger and alcohol. When you are in the Bowery, you're the lowest one can go. When men live under these poor conditions, they take on the characteristics of survival needed to live in the area. They also take on the label of "Bowery man" and the image of filth, drunkenness, worthlessness, and alienation it invokes. An image constantly reinforced as one steps over the bodies of other inhabitants or spends a lonely night in a 3x7 cube of a room.

It seems as if there are people that live like the men on the Bowery in every large city and every city has by necessity, design or history, a neighborhood to house the outcasts. But this grouping causes the area that is so selected to become a reinforcement hub for many of the ills of mankind. If perhaps such facilities were available that allowed the breaking up of the Bowery and spreading the rooming houses and shelters throughout the city, then the men might have an opportunity to divorce themselves from the stigma and the way of life they are often forced to live. In 1974 many men were trying.

Jim Boles, December 1974

September 2022 Update – The Skid Row is Gone

In September of 2022 I went back to the Bowery, forty-eight years after this paper was written. The 1970s buildings were there; the Salvation Army Booth House, the Bowery Mission, the bars, the One Mile House, the Majestic, and the Sunshine. The area looked like any lower Manhattan Street, the bars were gone, replaced with nice restaurants and stores, the flop houses were replaced with market-rate apartments, hotels, and condos. A few of the restaurant and lighting supply stores remained. I did not see many homeless men. New York has been gradually phasing out the concentration of men who were living in the Bowery starting later in the 1970's. They are trying to house the homeless in shelters and low-income housing, which is to some extent distributed in the city. The Bowery, the skid row of the 1970's is gone.

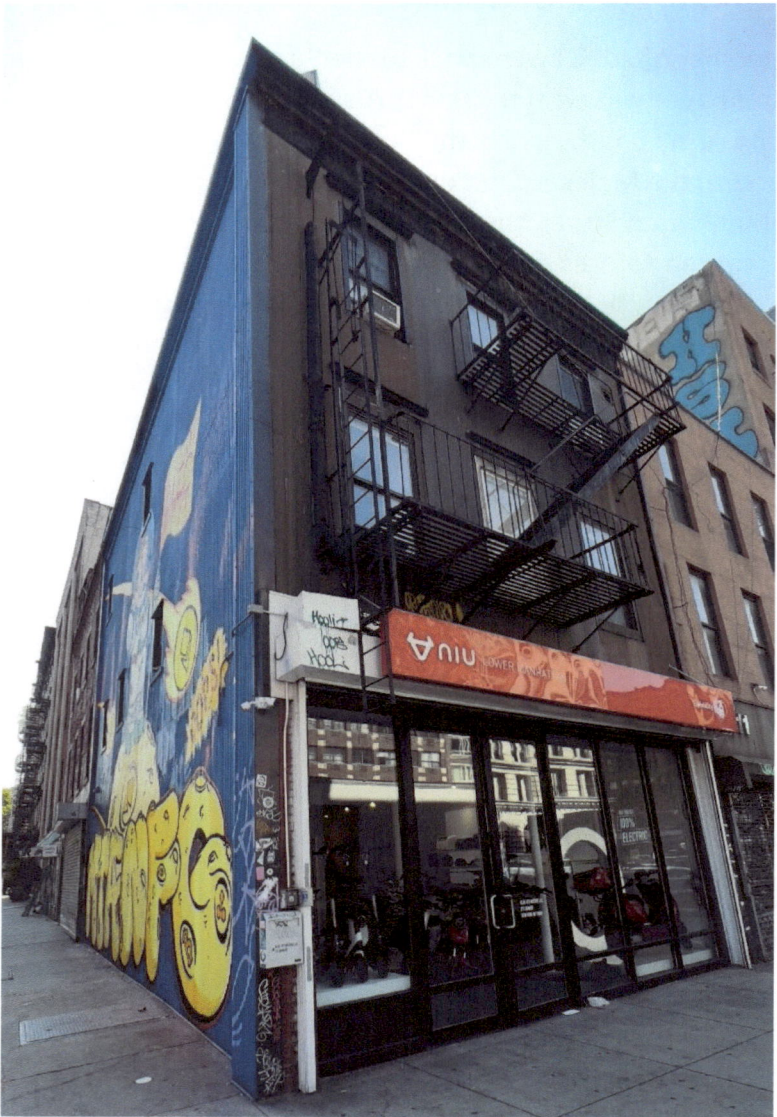

One Mile House Bar, 2022, photo by the author.
Now an electric scooter store.

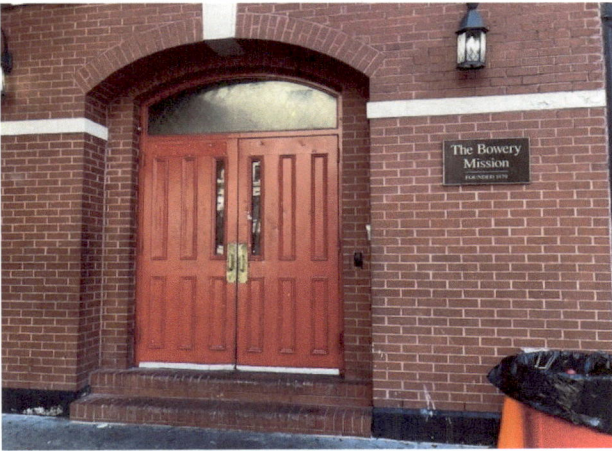

The Bowery Mission, 2022, photo by the author.

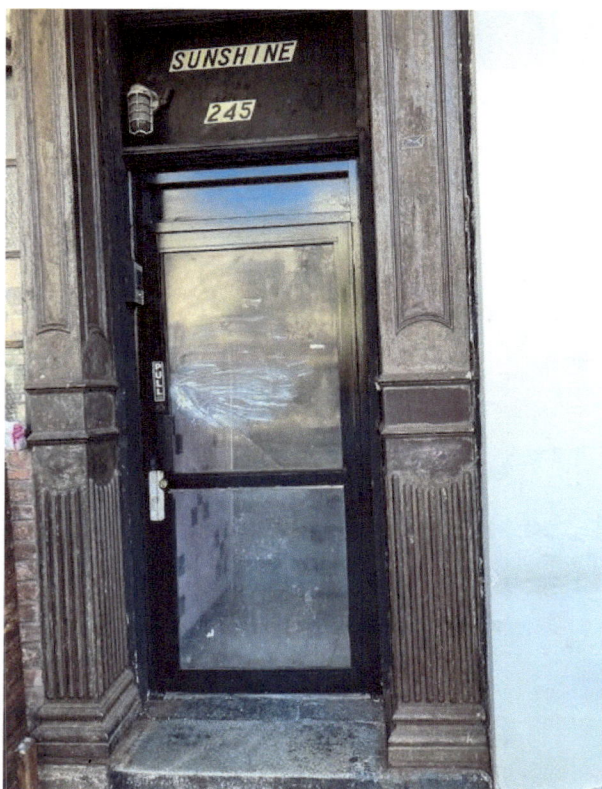

The Sunshine Hotel, 2022. Credit J. Boles.

Used in the Documentary Sunshine Hotel,
by Michael Dominic, 2001.

About the Author

James Boles, Ed.D, is a Lockport, New York, native, Army veteran, and retired CEO of People Inc., a Western New York health and human services organization. He received his doctorate in education from Columbia University. In 1998, he founded the Museum of disABILITY History, Buffalo, New York, receiving the Hervey B. Wilber Historic Preservation Award for his work with the museum. Under President George W. Bush, he was appointed for two terms on the President's Committee for People with Intellectual Disabilities. Now retired, Boles lectures and writes about the past. He has a strong interest in preserving history and promoting cultural tourism. This publication is one of a series that look at our past produced by Vanishing Past Press. The purpose of Vanishing Past Press is to encourage, develop, publish, and market works of scholarship and cultural importance, with a focus on under-examined and unexplored topics.

Additional References About the Bowery

The Bowery by Michael D. Zettler

Devil's Mile by Alice Sparberg Alexiou

On The Bowery, New York City, 1971 by Edward Grazda

Sunshine Hotel, Documentary, Michael Dominic, 2001, on Amazon Prime

Alcohol, a history by Rod Phillips

The Bowery Man by Elmer Bendiner

Flophouse, Life on the Bowery by Stacy Abramson and David Isay

Titles by Jim Boles

These books can be found at your local bookstore and Amazon.com.

No Harm was Done – Alternative Medicine in Niagara Falls, NY

Stories from the Springs – The Niagara Frontier. Also available in Ebook form

When There Were Poor Houses

Dr. Skinner's, Niagara Falls, New York School for "Colored Deaf and Dumb, and Blind Children" 1857

Cures and Care in Niagara County, New York 1830's-1950's

Ivan the Invacar Series: children's books, disability related.

The Gold Cure Institutes of Niagara Falls, NY

Contributed

On The Edge of Town: Almshouses of Western New York, -Publisher

No Offense Intended: A Directory of Historical Disability Terms, -Editor

Abandoned Asylums of New England: A Photographic Journey, by John Gray, -Publisher

Buffalo State Hospital: A History of the Institution in Light and Shadow, published by the Museum of disABILITY History, Buffalo, New York, - Publisher, editor

J.N. Adams Memorial Hospital – Her Inside Voice, by Char Szabo-Perricelli, published by the Museum of disABILITY History, Buffalo, New York, -Publisher, editor

Buffalo State Psychiatric Hospital: An Inside Report from the 1950s, by Patricia Kautz, published by the Museum of disABILITY History, Buffalo, New York, -Contributor

Path to the Institution: The New York State Asylum for Idiots, by Thomas E. Stearns – Executive Editor

Beautiful Childers: The Story of Elm Hill School and Home for Feebleminded Children and Youth, by Diana M. Katovirch, -Editor

Of Grave Importance: The Restoration of Institutional Cemeteries, by David Mack-Hardiman

www.ingramcontent.com/pod-product-compliance
Lightning Source LLC
Chambersburg PA
CBHW041229270326
41935CB00006B/60

9 781949 860030